Crohn's Disease

Living and Coping with it.

I0446779

Diary of an old Crohnie

A book designed to encourage self-help for people with Crohn's Disease, Colitis, and other Inflammatory Bowel Diseases, by reflecting on a real-life journey of a person who has been through it and is now sharing their experience.

.

Brian Prendergast

DEDICATION

Dedicated to my wife Geraldine and to 'Crohnies' all over the world.

This is a true-life account of the ups and downs, and my many different experiences and stories living with Crohn's Disease. I'm writing them so they may be used as a self-help guide for both people who have possibly just been diagnosed and are searching through the minefield of information on the internet, or for people who have a friend or relative who has the condition and are looking for help how to understand it all, so they may give some support and empathy.

The book is intended to be written with a lighthearted tone, but will tell of good times, and also some bad times. You might find it to be brutally honest at times, but at the end of it, I want you to take the good things from it and learn to avoid the bad. Everybody has different symptoms and levels of sickness, so the aim of this book is for 'All Crohnies' to learn to cope a bit better, by reading somebody else's story and knowing that you are not alone in this world.

Best of luck!

Brian Prendergast

CONTENTS

Introduction

Throughout the book I will be looking in at my own life, through self-reflection, and you may notice from reading this that a similar thing happened to you, or you can compare a certain stage in your life or can place yourself in a familiar situation.   These 'situations' or lifestyle choices were possibly one of the factors that lead to you becoming ill.   The exact cause of Crohn's Disease is still unknown. It can be something to do with genes, immune system, anxiety, smoking, depression, and digestive problems to name a few.

The hope is that if you can recognise the things that I went through, then you can make the necessary changes to get you better again.

This is not a medical book, it's more like a 'fly on the wall documentary' but written down in plain, understandable language.

For privacy I have changed some names of people and buildings mentioned in the book.

The child smoker

I am in primary school.   I am about 11 years of age.   Across the road is a newsagents / mini-mart.   Three of us go in with the equivalent of 5 cents.   We knew what to ask for, as the bigger lads in the school told us.   "A loose smoke and a match please".   We were handed a single cigarette and a red tipped match.   We lit it up and smoked it between us.   This became a regular occurrence, each one of us telling our mams on different days that we needed 5 cents for something in school.

The ironic thing is that this shop is now a funeral home!   It would end up taking me 30 years to give up putting a cigarette in my mouth.

Our Crohn's journey begins...

The early years

Our story begins in Merchants Arch, Dublin, Ireland.   This is a little archway that is across from Dublin's famous Halfpenny Bridge and leads up to Temple Bar.   Why was I there? Simply because it was the best busking spot in Dublin, as it was dry, shaded from the wind, and had a natural echo, similar to a mini concert hall.

1985 / 86 was the time of 'Live Aid', and Ireland's unemployment rate was massive. Things were so bad that somebody came up with the idea to have a concert in Dublin called 'Self Aid'.   Nobody could get a job.   Every second person was either heading to the USA or Australia.

They say one cause of Crohn's can be depression.   I think at that time, the whole of Ireland was depressed.   The music at the time was mostly rebellious, and when you went to gigs you would get in half price with your 'dole card' (welfare id).

Your Wednesday would consist of going into the welfare office in Gardiner Street. The floor tiles were done in such a way that they formed long lines, that would loop around to create a subliminal queueing system.

You would see the same fellas every week. You would end up at a hatch. Without even looking up at you, the clerk would say 'have you looked for work this week', you would say yes, and she would hand you a few quid and some butter vouchers. Butter vouchers you say? Yes, the EU had an overstock of butter, and they thought it would be a great idea to give it to the unemployed!

So, again you gave your mam a few quid, you had just about enough for a night in the pub with your mates, and the next morning you were broke again.

Essentially your stomach was always 'in a knot' because you were depressed. Depression is diagnosed quite quickly nowadays, but back then we were more than likely depressed but didn't know it!   We just had no job and not even the prospect of getting a job.   That went on for 18 months.   Every day the same, every week the same.   No wonder my stomach ended up in bits!

The chance of a job

Ireland at the time had a Government Training Agency called FAS, which after being a long time on welfare, they sent you to do a course that might get you a job.   So they sent me on one.   Electronic Assembly.   Now I thought this would be great, as even though they had just really been invented for the home market, I had a big interest in computers, and I still have my first one, a Sinclair ZX81 that my brother Gary bought for me when I was 12.

So I went in the first day of the course.   It turned out that it wasn't really an 'electronics' course, but more of an assembly course. Similar to putting pegs in boards, except you were doing it with ready made electronic parts. The good thing was I was getting paid for it, and it was double the rate on the 'dole'.   So I did it, and the instructor was great, and my fellow trainees were great and it was great to be learning something new, and having the prospect of a job at the end of it.   The course went on for 10 weeks, every day cycling downhill for about 3 miles, in hail, rain or sunshine. Problem was, on the way home it was 3 miles uphill. I reckon we didn't have global warming back then, because in the late 80's, it seem to lash rain every day!

So at the end of the 10 weeks, they sent us out to factories to try and find jobs. Well... It turns out that there were no jobs. These American companies were given all sorts of money to setup in Ireland, including being given buildings, if they stayed in Ireland for a minimum of 10 years. By this time, the 10 years was up, so they had shipped off their production to China or the Far East, and had just kept a minimal staff in Ireland.

We were going into huge buildings and warehouses, that only had about 15 people working in them, and I felt the only reason they were giving me an interview, was because they had to for some reason! So after the assumption and naivety of getting a job, there wasn't going to be one.   These companies had already seen their glory days, and were possibly getting funding just to keep going in Ireland, or for other reasons...

Bad and all that this sounds, it did help me when I was setting up my own company in later years.   But for the moment, I threw away my screwdriver!   The constant ups and downs of this time obviously played havoc with me. But it wasn't just me.   Everywhere you looked, every person you talked to.   People basically were in a bad state, and you either emigrated, or stayed and toughed it out.

Time for some drastic action

OK so at this point, I'm back on the dole like everybody else, and it's not looking great. So I spotted my brother Kevin's guitar in the corner.

Like so many others, he had gone to America to stay with my Uncle Martin and get a bit of work over there.

So I am now considering going busking. As a kid I had gone to piano lessons, and had always been into music, so I taught myself to play the guitar, but only a couple of chords. I was a bag of nerves but I headed off into town, into the place that at the time, and probably still is, the mecca for buskers – Grafton St. The only difference is nowadays, the buskers are usually doing it with guitars worth over a grand or more, amplifiers, microphones, and their lyrics on an iPad. There's no desperation here! It's more about getting likes and followers than needing a few quid to keep going!

So picture this... I am absolutely rattling. I have only 1 song, and I barely know the chords for it! Grafton St. has a little archway on it, that leads to a famous celebrity nightclub called Lillies Bordello. So I'm standing in this archway and have stepped back about 3 foot to keep out of the rain. McDonalds is right beside me. This is going to be great, lots of people passing by and I'm in out of the rain.

So I take the plunge, and start belting out 'American Pie' hoping there would be lots of tourists around. So after about half an hour, there is nothing in my guitar case that is on the ground in front of me. Not a red cent. So I'm determined, and I keep going, and I notice the odd person stopping at the side of the lane and then smiling at me and singing the song under their breath.

So after an hour, the rain had stopped, and there was 'nothing doing' so I decided to pack up and go home. It was at that moment that I had a revelation. No it wasn't a vision from above or a bolt of lightning.   It was just when I walked the 3 foot out into the street, that I spotted the 2 little fellas on each side of the entrance to the archway, that were hidden from my view, and had been shaking their McDonalds cups along to the music!   Worst part of all was their cups were full of coins!   At the time I was totally dejected, but when I look back on it, these kids were clever.   Good on them!

In the following weeks I stuck with the busking and moved to various spots around town. There was an unwritten etiquette amongst buskers that you only stayed in the 'good spots' for an hour, to give somebody else a chance, and then you moved on to a different one.

After about a year I ended up where this book begins, in Merchants Arch.   By this time, I had worked out a system.   I would look at people coming towards me in the distance and 'size them up'.   I now had 3 songs, American Pie if I thought they were American Tourists, Streets of London if they were English, and Summer in Dublin by Irish group Bagatelle if I thought they were Irish.   This worked out great and I wouldn't even sing the full song, unless they stopped to watch.   I'm sure there were shop owners in that area wondering who this guy is changing lyrics and songs midway, if he thought there were a couple of different nationalities going by!

New Job - The pressure begins

After 18 months of basically doing nothing, I was prepared to take any job, so on the 25th May 1987, I went for an interview for a job as a store man.   When I got there, the guy said, ahh sure I'm just looking for somebody to shift boxes the odd time, there's actually a friend of mine opening up around the corner, and he's looking for a salesman.   So he rang David in Banaman on Harcourt St. and sent me around and I got the job.

David would go on to become one of the few people I could call a lifelong friend, and we still are to this day, but Banaman turned out for me to be a mixed blessing.

The product was promotional items and mainly banners.   When I started to go out pounding the streets, I felt the shop owners and bar owners wouldn't listen to me, as I was only a young lad of 18.   David was a bit older, so we switched roles, he started selling and I started the manufacturing side of things.

I was great at the computer and was getting the best out of the equipment we had at the time. But what happened was, I became too good.

I was lashing stuff out really quickly, but unnecessarily. A customer would come in and maybe order a banner for a promotion they were doing next week. Being an eager young lad, I would have it done that day, even though it wasn't needed until next week.

I would do that with ALL of the orders. I would lie awake at night, knowing which job had to be done early as I had told the person it would be ready at a certain time.

Harcourt St. had little or no parking on it, so customers would sometimes 'double park' with their indicators flashing, and run in to collect their stuff. Problem was, sometimes it wouldn't be fully ready yet, and you had to keep chatting to them while running in and out to the back, waiting for the really slow printer to print the end of the banner, and then you had to laminate and trim it.

So if you're at this point in the book, and you're still wondering what this has to do with Crohn's Disease, well just look at what I was doing to myself.   And I MEAN doing to MYSELF.   The self-inflicted pressure I was putting myself under was crazy.   People just didn't expect their stuff that quickly.   It was purely myself being over zealous, hyper efficient, and proud of my work.

My body was on top form, but my stomach wasn't...

Problem was...I didn't see it coming...

With the odd pain in my side, I just ignored it, or maybe I just didn't want to see it coming, as I was way too dedicated to my job...

Day 1 of the rest of my life...

I can remember it today as clear as it happened then. I am on a hospital trolley in the emergency room. My dad has brought me in with a bad pain in my right side. My knees are up to my chest as that the only way of dealing with the pain. There is shouting and blood everywhere as there has been a 'razor fight' in Mountjoy Prison across the road. There are officers trying to hold down one prisoner, and my dad is using his body to shield me from the commotion.

I can hear 3 doctors talking in the corridor beside me. They think I have a bad appendix and it needs to come out. All 3 are complaining that they don't want to do it as they have been on 22 hour shifts. I am lying there saying 'oh great'. This is my first time ever in hospital. When I was a kid, I was amazed at the attention other kids got when they broke their arms with lots of people signing their 'plaster of Paris'. I always secretly wished I could go to hospital and get one of those!   Well, I got my wish.   I didn't think it would basically be in and out for the rest of my life!

Meanwhile my dad is talking to a nurse pointing at me, saying can you get a doctor for this fella NOW!

I feel a sharp pain in my side, and I pass out...

The Richmond Hospital

I wake up, and I'm in the Richmond Hospital. It is really old looking.   The nurses still wore the old fashioned head pieces that looked like something from World War 2.   You also had the matron dressed in black, who the nurses had to 'stand to attention' to whenever she walked into the room.

The beds actually really look like they are from back then.   They are the silver metal tubular type and have probably been hand painted about 50 times.

People are smoking in the ward.   I was a smoker at the time, and asked the guy in the next bed for a smoke.   He provided me with the essentials: a cigarette, a lighter, and the tin base off a Mr. Kipling cake (mini apple pie).

So back in those days, you could smoke in the ward, but get this, your visitors were allowed to smoke!   So when visiting time came, the hospital ward was a complete cloud.   It had more fog than a Duran Duran concert! Literally, you would not be able to see the end of the ward.

Sad thing was, you could smoke at any time! A fella would wake up in the middle of the night, and spark up a cigarette.   There would be little or no consideration for the guy in the bed next to him, the one on the oxygen tank!

They let me home about 4 days after the appendix operation with a small little scar down in that area.   I was still sore.

When I got home, I did bed rest, and started to eat again.

Within 2 days I was 'doubled up' in pain again, and was heading straight into the emergency department again.   This would be the first of many, hospital releases followed by taken straight back in again scenarios for the next couple of years.   In the emergency room they gave me an injection of some pain killer, and I was 'out for the count'.

The next morning I'm back in the same ward I was released from a couple of days ago.

One of the doctors that I remembered from the corridor the previous night came up to the side of my bed.

He was a young doctor and was genuinely emphatic to me. He said "when we took out your appendix, and we got it out before it burst".

So I'm thinking to myself – why is he looking so nervous? It was then he said to me that they "had done some tests and found evidence of Crohn's Disease".

"What?" I said, "were you able to get it sorted"? "No" he said, "it's an incurable disease". Well... You can imagine the cursing and swearing out of me...

What the F is Crohn's Disease?

Here I am, a young lad of about 18, after being told I now had an incurable disease!   What's going through my head is – I'm dying! (Obviously not!)

I'm thinking, they must have made a complete mess of my appendix operation as they were over-tired etc., and I genuinely thought that for weeks, but of course it wasn't true.

Nobody, and I mean Nobody, had ever heard of Crohn's Disease, or Crohn's as it's now shortened to, probably to make breaking the news to a patient a bit easier for the doctor!

In people's head, disease meant cancer, and incurable meant terminal!   That's not the case, but when you tell new people about it, you know that's what they are thinking.

Everybody is different and it affects people in different ways, and at different levels, so all I can do is quote the Mayo Clinic, as my opinion would be just based on my own experience.

"Crohn's disease is a type of inflammatory bowel disease (IBD). It causes swelling of the tissues (inflammation) in your digestive tract, which can lead to abdominal pain, severe diarrhea, fatigue, weight loss and malnutrition".

"Inflammation caused by Crohn's disease can involve different areas of the digestive tract in different people, most commonly the small intestine. This inflammation often spreads into the deeper layers of the bowel".

"Crohn's disease can be both painful and debilitating, and sometimes may lead to life-threatening complications".

"There's no known cure for Crohn's disease, but therapies can greatly reduce its signs and symptoms and even bring about long-term remission and healing of inflammation. With treatment, many people with Crohn's disease are able to function well".

*Source – MayoClinic.org 2023

I remember one doctor gave me a simple explanation to tell people if they asked me.

You put your food down your mouth, and it ends up in your intestine. Just imagine your intestine is like a garden hose. If there was a narrowing in the hose, then water would slow down and possibly get backed up. In my case, a section of the intestine would become inflamed, and any food trying to get through it would cause severe pain.

So again after about 2 weeks of a hospital stay, they let me out on tablets called Deltacortril, as they were reluctant to operate on such a young person. At one point, I am on 32 tablets a day, to be decreased as we go on.

Another hospital in – out. The Richmond was to become a revolving door...

Back to work - barely

I am now at home, and taking the 'Deltas' and and painkillers. At the moment it's jut the little scar, and I've read in books, that getting over an appendix operation is reasonably quick. Yes, books. The internet hadn't really caught on yet! So I am eager to get back to work, as in my head I think my boss can't cope on his own with the manufacturing (of course he could) so I went back probably earlier than I should.

It was great to be back. But that pain in my side was getting worse, as we decreased the tablets. I thought it would be going away, and it hadn't really sunk in that I had this Crohn's thing they were talking about.

Part of my job involved using a heat press for printing t-shirts, and let's say it wasn't the most modern one, so to clamp it down, you literally had to hang out of the thing! This wasn't a great idea, as along with the self imposed stress of getting orders out quickly, and keeping customers happy, this thing was using my stomach muscles.   Added to lifting boxes etc., I wasn't going to last long.

I lasted about a month, and I was back in the emergency room...

The many tests begin...

So I'm now in hospital again and the staff are beginning to become on first name terms with me. They are deciding that they are going to plan surgery for me. But before surgery, you've got to do all the tests! They have me on pain meds while they decide what they are going to do.

These were the first time I had ever had any of these tests, and I can tell you now, they were the first of many.

So apart from the obvious xrays and urine samples, one of my first references to poo is the stool test. Crohn's and IBD in general is all about poo, so there will be plenty of references to it. I'm calling it poo because if I use the word beginning with S, it might affect the book some way.

Anyway the stool test involved you doing a poo into a chair with a basin under it called a commode. Now here's the embarrassing part, you have to remember this is the old Richmond Hospital.   There are about 12 beds to a ward. You can't walk to the toilet, as you've a pain in your side and you're bed ridden.

The nurse wheels in the commode and roars at the top of her voice: "Now Brian, see if you can do anything for me in that now, won't ya."

The nurses back then all seemed to be farmers daughters from the country used to dealing with cattle and pigs, no bother to them.   They would ALWAYS roar instructions at you, even if you were right beside them, and embarrassingly roar out your conditions or symptoms.

This is the truth when I say one of them asked me one day – "did your bowels move today"? Now I had never ever heard that expression before.   Did your bowels move!   So I'm thinking it must be that sound your tummy makes when you're hungry like a rumbling bubbly sound, so of course I said no.   She would come back later and ask, did your bowels move in the afternoon Brian?   And again I would say no, and I actually remember saying to her, well I might have done one in my sleep, but I didn't really notice it.   This went on for about 3 days!   Little did I know it was simply asking did you do a poop.

Well they had me on every laxative known to man, including my dad bringing in his 'old wives tail cure' – Prune Juice, and made me drink the bottle of it!

Hence they wanted a stool test, so we're back in the ward, that big open ward, with about 12 beds.   The only separator between myself and the rest of the 'sick audience' is a thin curtain, that the nurse has forgotten to close properly!

Well, I felt the rumblings from within like as if you've just unblocked a drain, they had literally opened the flood gates.   I broke wind that sounded like the Titanic leaving the harbour! The waft carried down the whole ward, and you could hear the grunts of displeasure as it reached each nostril on the way down.   This carried on for about 24 hours, and God love the people on the ward, some of them were on oxygen masks!

Each time, the nurse would come down with a chart with little pictures of poops. Small ones, big ones, thin ones, fat ones, slushy ones, and then a cross section of all of them! She would then put a tick against which one you had just produced, and put it in the file to show the doctor. That was the stool test!

I know we're starting to get a bit graphic here, but these things were, and are, a reality for us Crohnie's, but your mates think this is all hilarious when you tell them! I'll be honest and say this humour helped me get through the whole thing, as you can laugh about it or cry, and it's a lot better to laugh.

Put it this way, as a Crohnie, your medical discussions and explanations to your mates, for the rest of your life is going to be about poo and farts, regularity, consistency, and velocity!

Another test that was done almost every time was a Barium Meal. So when you're first told about this test, you are visualising a foreign food, maybe Moroccan or something, as I had never heard of this before.

No it's not a meal at all, I wonder why they call it meal? Basically you are asked to swallow about a litre of this pink chalky liquid, but you couldn't really called it a liquid, maybe nearer to a milk shake consistency.

The idea of this is that as the drink goes down your throat, into your stomach and intestines, it glows under x-ray, and can show up pin holes, or inflammation, or other stuff, so the surgeon knows exactly where to go, when you're getting an operation.

The downside of this, is they can't leave all that stuff in your body if you're sick. In a 'normal' person, it would pass through 'naturally' over a couple of days, but in my case it was always followed by an 'Enema', which was basically getting 'flushed out' to encourage you to empty your bowel.   In my case, this would make me weak, and delay surgeries as I was too weak to undergo surgery.

This is one of the reasons my hospital stays were long, is because they would not give you any food just 'in case' the doctor wanted to do something with you.   Then by the time the doctor has decided what to do, you've to do the Barium Meal.   Then they flush you out with the Enema, and by the time you have had your surgery done, you are like a rag doll!

Then when you can't eat anything for a while after the surgery, while its repairing.   The final obstacle is that they can't let you home as you need to gain some weight!

So after years of this, I had my post surgery system worked out.   Double milky breakfasts and treble desserts instead of dinner to start. Fattened you up in no time!   For rapid weight gain my local doctor put me on a milk shake type drink called Ensure Plus.   Not Ensure, but instead Ensure Plus.   Bingo!   Did the job!

Gone Fishin...

OK, so now they have me 'cleaned out' internally, after several 'volcanic eruptions', its time for another test. – The scope.

So the doctor comes in, and casual as can be says, "we're going to take a sample of your bowel to see how things are down there". So I said "is this an operation"? "No" said he, "you'll be awake while we're doing it".

So I said to myself, this can't be too bad. However I did notice some of the other men in the ward grinning as the porter was wheeling me down...

So we end up in this room in the hospital marked Endoscopy, and they lay me up on the table. I'm expecting that they are going to do a small incision, or something keyhole to take a sample of my bowel.

Next thing he produces this thing that looked like a cross between a policeman's truncheon and a fishing rod!

"OK, bend over and bring your right knee up to your chest". Well... Talk about singing soprano? You'd want to hear the language out of me. The 'rod' has a camera on the end of it, that helps the doctor guide a 'mini scissors' to snip off a tiny piece of infected bowel for a test. But the operator had to twist it to get the right angle. All I was short of doing was smiling for the camera! It would have been hard to smile for anything, as I remember on my first one, biting into the nurse's sleeve of her cardigan!

That was back then. Back then they didn't give you any pre-meds, it was a real ahh sure get on with it, but nowadays they do, so you just feel a little 'happy'. There is no actual pain getting an endoscope, it's more just a 'strange' sensation when you get it for the first time. The equipment has changed now, so it's much easier and some people go back to work straight after it. Sometimes they use the scope to go down via your mouth, so I hope it's washed regularly!

My first operation...

They are now planning for my first surgery. The main doctor comes in, followed by about 10 junior doctors, each one shuffling to get to the front so they can hear him.

He proceeds to place his hand extremely gently on the appendix scar area, and tells the others that "Mr. Prendergast has a 'Crohn's mass' here. Is it ok Mr. Prendergast if my students examine you"? I agreed... I shouldn't have! These 10 idiots started leaning full force with the palm of their hands on the sore area. "I can't feel it, can you? Yes, it's right there". They were literally arguing with themselves for about 15 minutes while each one of them had a go!

The operation was delayed by a week, as I was now too sick to get it done, because of these fools! The same thing happened me a couple of years later, where I was due to get out, and they came in to show the students how one of the operations went. They leaned on me so hard, that they caused me a massive amount of pain, and I distinctly remember being kept on for a further 2 weeks because of that.

So we're back to my first operation, it was a bowel resection.   Ok, we're going to imagine the garden hose again.   Just imagine there's 2 kinks in it.   They cut out the length of hose that has the kinks, and join the 2 fresh bits of hose together.   The problem is sometimes, where they stitch those 2 pieces together can become inflamed, and they have to go again.

There was no keyhole surgery back then, well not in The Richmond anyway!   I was cut from just above my groin area, circled around my belly button, and up to just below my chest. Nice cut.   The lads were well impressed!   An epic war wound for future years!

Problem was, every time I would have a surgery, they would go through the same cut, so it always took a long time to heal.

All in all I was in and out The Richmond for

about a year, with the longest continuous stretch being 3 months. They had put me in a ward with 2 other young guys, Dessie from Letterkenny in Donegal, and Justin from Dublin. Dessie had got shingles that went into his spine, and after initially walking into the ward, he ended up in a wheelchair when his condition worsened. Justin had damaged his back some way, and was getting bits of metal put into it. We were all 'long stayers' so by the end of 3 months we had the run of the place. Getting a TV and Video Player brought in from home, ordering Four Star Pizza via the back door of the hospital, it was like we had our own apartment.

One day they moved Justin to a different part of the hospital across a little road called The Hardwicke Unit. Well of course Dessie thought it would be a great idea to go over and visit Justin if I pushed him in the chair. So talk about the blind leading the blind, we went over. Problem was, we stayed too late, and the gates to the main hospital were closed. So

I'm pushing Dessie, with a scar the length of my belly, and meant to be getting out soon. Luckily there was a gap in the railings and I was able to squeeze through and stand him up and squeeze through also. But the chair wouldn't fit. It wasn't a collapsible one. So I lifted it and threw it over the gate. Well you would want to see the 2 of us trying to sneak back into the hospital via service entrances and nearly knocking over several gas tanks on the way! We got in, and said nothing. Next morning, the porter was confused by the state of the buckled wheels on the chair that he has just brought him up the day before. "How the hell did that happen"? "Ehh... No idea!"

Anyway there was several 'ins and outs' but I eventually went back to Banaman on a walking stick for the first week as I was still a bit weak. They had taken on two extra people while I was out, so it was strange, because they had come into the company with nobody there, and suddenly there was me. It caused a bit of worry at the time - not good for Crohn's.

3rd patient in Beaumont Hospital...

The Richmond Hospital was closing down (it's now a court house), and it was merging with Jervis St. Hospital. They were merging into Beaumont hospital, which had been built five years earlier, but had been lying empty since then over 'red tape arguments' or something.

The Richmond still had patients (namely me) and for the big press launch and pulling back the curtain on the plaque, they had decided to take the eldest person from The Richmond, and the eldest person from Jervis St. to be the first patients in the new hospital.

There was a massive motorcade of ambulances that had been drafted in from all over the country, for this almost military operation!

I just happened to be in the third ambulance! So the first two ambulances had the two old ladies, Charlie Haughey our prime minister at the time, met them at the doors, and brought them over to the plaque wall. He shook hands with me as I passed by, as they were bringing me straight in, as the ladies were busy getting press photos done.   So technically you could say I was the first person to actually get into the hospital, but I will give that credit to the two ladies.

The first thing I notice is that this place is spotless, and I mean spotless.   The Richmond had two sisters as cleaners, one with black hair and the taller one blonde.   They were about 50 to 60 at the time, and had been there for years.   They had to kneel down and polish the wooden floor.   It was only in later years, they got buffers.   The sisters used to let us smoke and make tea for ourselves in their little area. Every evening after their shift, the oul matron would come along with a white linen handkerchief and run her finger around the edges of the doors and corners.   If there was even the slightest hint of dirt, they were made do it again.

But Beaumont was new.   Straight out of the

wrapper!   There was about 6 to a ward, and each ward had a 'common room' with a telly, and lovely armchairs, and you could smoke, in the room, and it also had a balcony.

I was now on tablets called Prednisolone, they were steroids, and as every crohn's patient is different, they didn't work for me.   So after another snip of intestine out of me, and through the same scar, I was sent home on those tablets and pain killers.

Sad thing was I went back for an out patient appointment six months later, the common room was filthy!   It was literally filthy with cigarette burns in the armchairs and on the carpet.   All you could smell was ash on the balcony.   I was really shocked to see how something can be wrecked in such a short time.   They then closed it.

It's a pity, and I know nowadays that they keep that hospital spotless again, but unfortunately Beaumont has the highest rate of hospital bug in Ireland...   *Source Irishtimes.com/health/2022/12/27/

I meet my saviour – both of them...

I've gone a good few months feeling ok now, so it's Halloween Night about 1988. Myself and the lads decide to go to a night club in The Phoenix Park Racecourse, called The End. We had been going there for a while, and knew that this night was fancy dress. So I went as Crocodile Dundee in a hat with corks hanging out of it, big boots, green safari shorts, and a Hawaiian shirt.

I spotted this little beauty across the dancefloor, and there was three of them, and none were in fancy dress. They had been in the pub across the road and had only decided to come in at the last minute.

Anyway I gave her a couple of winks across the dancefloor and she kept laughing at me, so as soon as the 'slow set' came, I was over like a rocket.

She was (and still is) absolutely gorgeous, and when she told me she worked in a supermarket, I told her I would make her a namebadge (from Banaman).   Anyway we went home separate ways, but we had a mutual friend Linda, that worked across the road.   So the next day, I lashed out a namebadge in work, and dropped it into Linda in her house, along with an envelope with my phone number on it.

Nothing for a week...   Never turned up to The End...   I was gutted.   After two weeks, Linda went over to Geraldine's shop for something, and said "oh yes! I actually have something for you"!   Ger looked at the namebadge, and phoned me.   We were married two years later, I was aged 20 and she was 22.   But we knew right then that we were destined for each other and so far are Thirty Three years happily married.   She was my first saviour, as without Geraldine, I may not have got through some of the things still to come.

The second saviour was a lot different, and some of you readers can take this at face value of what happened and how it affected me.

My mam and dad brought us up as Catholics, but weren't strict about it at all. You would pretend to go to mass, but really you'd be outside chatting to your mates having a smoke.

Mam had heard from a 'friend of a friend' that there is this religious artefact, a relic of the true cross, kept under lock and key in the non public area of Church St. Church, near Dublin City.

She hoped that it might heal me, so I went along with the process for her sake. She had to make an appointment with the priest, and the way this relic worked was you had to bring the whole family.

I remember it exactly as it happened. We were brought into a side room and were asked to sit around this large table. The priest then produced a red velvet bag, and out of it came the most beautiful cross you've ever seen. It had a glass dome in the centre with a miniature blue silk cushion, and on the cushion was a splinter.   The priest told us it was brought to his order of priests a very long time ago, and nobody knows the exact date, but early 1600's they have a record of it coming from abroad.   The splinter is supposed to be splinter from the true cross, or in other words, the cross that Jesus died on.

While he is saying this to us, I can see out of the corner of my eye, my brother Kevin grinning at my brother Gary trying to make him laugh with this 'waffle'.

Anyway the priest asked us to join hands, and starting saying a prayer that was with the cross.   We all had our eyes closed but he held the cross over my head.

It was at that point that I experienced a feeling that I had never felt before.   It was a 'magnetic' feeling that was pulling me upwards towards the cross.   I obviously made a sound because the others opened their eyes.   They said at the time that my face was glowing red with happiness.   I stayed quiet.   Mam asked me had I any pain, and my answer was no...   I stayed quiet the whole way home...   I was lucky to have two more similar experiences in later years, that I will tell you about later.   As I said at the start of it, all I can do is tell you what happened, but I got a long break from the illness after that...

I join the band...

Months started to go by and I was feeling well.
I was on new tablets called Salazopyrin which
is essentially an anti-inflammatory drug,
designed to keep the flare ups at bay. I was
back in Banaman, I loved it, and I loved making
different things every day. We used to do
promotional items for large events, and it was
great to see the banner you printed on the
newspaper, or teams in an event with your t-
shirts on.

Myself and Ger used to meet up after work
and go into a pub around the corner on
Camden St. / Wexford St. called The Vintage.
It was great for making toasted sandwiches, so
you could soak up the beer, and keep going for
a few more hours.

I knew my Uncle Jimmy (by marriage) played in
a ballad group called Gypsy Rovers, and played
in a pub right across the street. So we went
over half drunk one night, and there I am
telling Ger that was my Uncle right there for

the whole night through beer goggles.   It turned out to be a different band altogether called Gypsy Lacey!   I hadn't seen Jimmy in a while but I remembered he had a beard, and this guy did too.   (Frankie – Gypsy Lacey).   We eventually got to a real gig, and we thought they were great.

It turned out their guitarist was leaving! Jimmy was always an awful worrier, and tended when anybody left the band to grab the first person available.   He had known I had done the busking and played the guitar, so I was really lucky that I was the one he had his sights set on.

So we arranged a practice session in my garage.   You had Martin, Jimmy and Red and myself.   Jimmy later told me that Red was anxious of the fact that I was so young, and I might leave the band to go off and join a rock band or something, but I loved Irish music, and had listened to my dad singing in Pubs all my life.   After being able to match the speed of

Reds banjo playing I was accepted into the band.   Red later went off to become a Principal Teacher in a school in Mayo, but myself, Martin and Jimmy, are now 34 years playing together which we will talk more about later, as we all went our separate ways for a while.

The band was a release for me creatively, but also caused me stress and anxiety, as again I was a perfectionist, and this time it wasn't customers, it was the crowd in The Wexford Inn I wanted to keep happy by bringing in new songs.   Again, this was completely self-imposed, as some bands got away with playing the exact same set for years, but some of you 'crohnies' will recognise this personality trait of just wanting to keep everybody happy and doing the best you can do.

One evening we were playing in a pub called The Stillorgan Orchard.   I had felt a bit of a pain in my side but put it down to food.   Half way through the gig we would always take a 15 minute break. We used to say we were taking a wee break, but we were really taking a 'wee wee' break to go to the toilet!

I went out to the car park and was doubled up in pain. An ambulance was called. I was taken to St. Vincents hospital on the south side of Dublin. The remission was over... I was back in again...

St. Vincent's Hospital...

Back in the day, hospitals used to take turns in being 'on call'. This meant the emergency rooms in various hospitals around the country would be the one on duty for accidents etc.

On that night the Mater Hospital on the north side of the city and St. Vincent's on the south side were on call. The ambulance did not give you a choice. They went to the nearest one, and St. Vincent's was the nearest to the pub, so I ended up there.

It was old but more modern. The smoking in the wards was gone at that stage but you could still smoke at the end of the corridor. When smokers went into hospital at that time, all they were concerned about is 'where can you smoke'. Their leg could be hanging off, but they were still more concerned about smokes!

Over the years, I did have some stays in the Mater, but they would be short, as they always wanted you to stick with the hospital and team you had always been dealing with, so they would switch me back to Beaumont.

But this place St. Vincent's was MILES away from my home!   Ger didn't drive at the time, and would have to get two buses out to it. Sometimes I would be so whacked out on painkillers, that I would be asleep when she got there and didn't want to wake me. Sometimes she would just go home, but sometimes she would wait hours till I came around.   Unbelievable.

My mother used to do the same.   God love her, again taking two buses, it was about a four hour round trip.   Then to get there, and I've been taken down for a test, or just completely whacked!   My Dad would come in on his way home from work, but it must have been very disheartening for them sometimes.

St. Vincent's at the time turned out to be the main hospital in Ireland dealing with Crohn's and had both the number one surgeon and physician at the time.   They asked me did I want to switch my care over from Beaumont to them and of course I said yes.

St. Vincent's turned out to be more in's and out's but on a bigger scale.   This time I was a bit older, and able to cope with things a bit better, but the operations began to get bigger, and the stays would be longer.   The short stays would never be less than two weeks, but the longer stays would be three months.

My boss David kept my job open the whole time...

Operations get bigger...

The next operation was called an Extended Right Hemicolectomy. When they were telling me this, they might as well have been telling me anything, or speaking in a foreign language.

Unfortunately doctors in hospital have to do large rounds (get around to a lot of people). They never talk to you, they talk to the junior doctors beside them, to advise them what to do with you.

In later years, I would speak up for myself, and stop the main doctor, and get him to explain in basic English exactly what the plan is. I think they respected me for that. After all, at this stage, my file was the thickness of the 'Yellow Pages', and today we are on the third one of those, reason why – later.

So this Extended Right Hemicolectomy is basically more intestine and other bits being taken away. But...whilst they were 'in there', they would spot another bit that was inflamed, and take that away also.   So this is one of the reasons for the long stays.   I would be just over one surgery and I would have to get another.

This particular one was a good example, as when they opened me up (again through the same scar) it left the skin around the centre of my chest bone a bit thin.   This caused a hernia, where a piece of bowel, intestine, whatever you like to call it, would rest against this area, and become trapped causing a 'bubble' on the surface.   Basically a bit of bowel trying to get out!

So on that occasion, I was wheeled back down again, opened up (again through the same scar) and they put a piece of mesh inside me to form let's say a thicker barrier, that the bowel wouldn't get lodged in it.   I had suggested to them that while they're doing next one, they can put a zip in the scar!

St. Vincent's was also a University hospital, and they used to have the top surgeons and physicians from around the world attending 'Crohn's' conferences. I was that long there, and they knew me so well, that they used to wheel me down and use me as a lecture piece.

One of the times I actually asked the organizing doctor could I address the crowd...and I did. My wife came and I addressed the hall of about 200 top guys in the world, and basically pleaded with them to get their heads together, and use each other's knowledge, and find some sort of cure for this damn condition.

You would want to see me. At this point I was in a wheelchair as my legs were weak from severe weight loss. They FAST you for everything in hospital, for almost every test, no matter how small, so you lose weight very quickly. Then the struggle is to get it back on!

But that day, I made the decision to fight, and I let them know that I wanted them to fight also. It actually worked! They offered me a place to go on a clinical trial that was going on worldwide, and there was going to be a handful of patients from Ireland.

A clinical trial for example is where out of 100 patients that are sick, they will give 50 of them the actual drug, and the other 50 will get a tablet that looks the exact same, but is probably just sugar.   The patients symptoms / recovery are monitored, and they can tell whether the drug is having an effect or not. The fake one is called a 'placebo' drug.

It's also used to monitor side effects.   If you had a headache, and I gave you a white pill containing sugar, and your headache was gone after 10 minutes, and your hair starts falling out.   You can't blame me for your hair falling out, as you were given sugar, the fake one!

I ended up turning down the clinical trial, as I personally couldn't face getting my hopes up and then finding out I was given the fake one.

That drug went on to become 'Remicade'.   A known treatment for Crohn's Disease.

All good – for a while...

In the meantime, my two fantastic twins were born, Anthony and Christina. I was getting a break from surgeries for a good while, and the Salazopyrin seemed to be working.

So I needed to start to earn a few quid extra. I couldn't ask my boss for anything else after him keeping my job open all those times, but I needed to upskill myself, so I could make more money for Banaman, then I could possibly earn more. I had been pestering David for a computer for years. Computers were relatively new at the time, and we were still doing our design on a dot matrix printer, and enlarging logos using a photocopier, using a black felt tip pen to smoothen out the edges.

I was on my lunch break on Baggot St. Dublin, and I spotted this large sign over a café – Computer Training and on the list was Computer Graphics and Desktop Publishing. I started that week. The course was run by Pat and the teacher was Trevor. On one side of the desk was three Macs, and on the other side was three PC's. So this training company was way beyond it's time, as in the graphic design game, you have to learn the software on both systems, as some companies use Mac's and were 'die hard' mac fans, whereas others used PC's which were about half the price.

I was in my element here. I was bringing the stuff I had designed into David, constantly trying to tease him into finally getting a computer.

Pat sat in on some of the classes. When the course was over, Pat said to me something like "you were really good at that, did you ever consider teaching it"? I told him I had given guitar lessons in the past, and that was about it! He gave me the course notes and curriculum for the City and Guilds courses he was planning to run. Possibly somebody had let him down, but I was in the door and teaching those classes within a week in the evenings after Banaman.

After a while CT took off really well and moved to a larger building on Fitzwilliam Square. It was brilliant. I was upskilling for free! Pat would have me sit in on a course for free as a student, and then suddenly I would be teaching it. He was getting an enthusiastic teacher, and I was getting City and Guilds qualifications, which held importance at that time. I was the graphics guy, and the beginners classes guy, but as I sat in on more courses, I also became the stand in guy when any of the other teachers went on holidays etc.

One time we ran a City and Guilds Computer Hardware course. I had sat in on this one and loved it, but it was so popular we needed two teachers. I had now convinced David to buy that computer as I could get it cheaper via CT, as we could build it from scratch.

Pat sat me down one evening and went through step by step, how to assemble and setup this computer. I was hooked! I had messed around with stereos and amplifiers before, but this was a computer! It's spec was Windows 3.1, 2 mb ram and 40mb hard drive, and that was fast at the time! You will realise later on how important this moment was.

So now we had a mortgage, two kids, and I had come to the realisation that I was working in Banaman during the day, was working as an Adult Computer Trainer for two nights of the week, and was playing gigs in The Wexford Inn on Saturdays with the band.

I did this for a couple of years, but something was going to 'give way' at some stage. There was no way I could keep that up, but it was the same old story. Making as much as you can whilst you're well, and saving for the bad times.

It did give way!...

Everything gone...

A couple of years had passed. In quite a short space of time the rock fall happened. After working in my first real job for over 12 years, I had to say goodbye to Banaman. There were so many 'in's and outs' and massive amounts of time off recovering, that there was no way we could continue on. Add to the fact, that although I loved the job, the self-imposed pressure and stress was killing me, so we finished on great terms.

Around the same time, CT had become a lot bigger and was running day courses along with evening. The demand for graphics courses had gone down, and although Pat actually offered me a full time job, I couldn't tell him at the time that I would never have been able to take it, so CT went away for a while.

Then I also had to leave the band, as I would get weak at gigs, as we had got to the stage where sometimes we were playing 3 or 4 nights a week, with 90% of them being for charity or friends.   Again I left on great terms as they knew I wasn't able for it at that time.

So everything happening all at once.   It had it's toll on my body, and where did I end up?   Of course...back in St. Vincent's.

In a very short time everything had just 'hit the fan' and my biggest challenge was still yet to come...

Reflection...

Before I start this section, I would like to say that if this experience ever happened to me again, I know I would handle it a lot better, but at the time, for a young man with two young kids, and bills to pay, it was very tough. If you the reader are going through it, then by reading this, take it from me, you WILL get through it...

We are back in the usual ward in the usual corridor. At this point, the smoking in the corridors was gone, so you sneaked down in the lift to the car park, even if you had a drip stand with you.

This time I am very sick. I have gone down to eight stone (112 lbs), and for about a 28 year old man, meant to be in the prime of his life, this is very underweight. My body is what's known as emaciated. This is where after rapid weight loss, the skin of my belly was 'empty' and sagging over the rest of my body. All skin was loose.

On my arms, where once was muscle, is now swaying skin. My eyes were sunken into the back of my head, and I genuinely looked like somebody from a famine starved part of the world.

Again we had the usual rounds of fasting – then a test – then fasting again, whilst they figure out what they are going to do.

After the tests, they told me that they had found a lot of inflammation this time, and would have to take out multiple pieces.

They then told me they might have to do an 'Ileostomy'. According to Mayo Clinic - an ileostomy is usually done to the small bowel, whereas a colostomy usually deals with the large bowel. I never had a colostomy, so I won't talk about it, but yes I can talk about the ileostomy. Once again I will say that if I was told I was to have this again, I would cope a lot better now, between hindsight, and life experiences. I would definitely cope better today. Back then wasn't the case...

The Big One...

I woke up after the surgery. The immediate first thing that went through my head was 'did they do the bags'? I was in the recovery room, and I was still whacked out on meds, and I spotted Geraldine in the corner. They had never let her into that area before, so I had a feeling that something was up. I beckoned her over, and although I couldn't really speak, I pointed to my belly area. She said yes you've got the bags, and said but they're ok, they're grand. I knew she was just trying to save face and cheer me up. They had done an ileostomy, I now had two bags on my stomach area.

They had basically cut the intestine, and brought the two ends to the skin surface of my stomach / belly area, cut a hole, and poked them through. The one on my right side was small, more like a pouch and a clear sticky substance came out of it. This was probably some sort of mucus type liquid the bowl produces to help your food slide down, but this side was to have no food going through it, so obviously the mucus type sticky stuff just came of this side.

The one coming out my left side was the bag, about 12 inches long, that stuck onto your skin to cover the 'stoma' (the bit of my inside that was now sticking out of my body).   The bag had a suction collar that was meant to stick, but it was a nightmare.   This was 30 years ago, I hope they have decent ones now!

So this particular bag was what my body was going to poop into for the next six months.   It had a special clip at the end of the bag, and you would go into a toilet, open the clip, and let it fall down into the bowl and flush.   The doctors had told me that it was going to be a temporary one, and the operation would be reversed in six months time.   From day one I was waiting for the six months to end.   Instead of my bum, my poop, and farts, were going into this bag!   I am still peeing the normal way.

Two nights after I'm in the hospital bed going to sleep. They had started me on light desserts and yoghurts etc. to get my system working again. I woke up at about 3 am. My bed was wet. I turned on the light and my bed was destroyed, the bag had come off. I had said that the bags had a circular collar on them, that was made of a synthetic rubber that as you heated it more with your body heat, it was meant to stick longer. Mine didn't and this was the first of many times, that I would have 'adult accidents', stop laughing, yes I was like a big baby, but yes, these damn things gave me MANY adult accidents at the start.

The thing was, whoever decided to stick my stoma out of my body to the outside, didn't do it on a flat area. They placed near the crease just below my belly where you bend down! Absolutely disastrous place to put it, but its possible it was the only place half suitable. So every time I either bent down, or brought my knees up, the thing would come off! It was at this time I met a senior nurse called Sister G and this person is what I would call a human angel! I was being kept in the hospital because I was still recovering from the surgery, but they wanted to make sure I was 'mentally' accepting the bags. Well as I said to them hundreds of times, of course I am 'mentally' accepting the bags, but the effing things keep coming off and destroying the place, that's what has me 'not mentally' pooing all over the place!

Well... Sister G was the person you would call the Crohn's nurse nowadays, that most hospitals have now, and she literally took me under her wing. We starting trying the white tape the nurses use to stop you bleeding after injections, and put tape all around the edges.

She contacted the manufacturers of the bags for any tips. She got me samples of different brands of bags to try. Sometimes the bag would stay on but the clip at the end of the bag would fail, so she sourced different types of clips. She took a genuine interest in me and gave me care that was really needed at the time. One other issue the bags had was being a bit small and filling up too quicky. If you had a bowl of soup, then almost the whole bowl of soup would end up in that bag. So you had the weight of the liquid pulling the bag off the side of you, and if it didn't stick, then it's Niagra Falls again!

I then remember, from one of her many enquiries, she came up with this belt little plastic hooks on it that held up the weight of the bag and took the pulling away part out of the equation. This worked really well!

So with the circular suction thing, some glue that Sister G had come up with, that helped stick it to my skin, rolls of tape, and this hook belt, and my little addition – we now had a system that worked! My idea, was once we had all the other bits done, I would put on tight fit cycling shorts over the whole lot, and the compression of the shorts held everything in place, then trousers over the whole lot.

So they let me out and I hoped these things would stay on. For me it was rough getting to this stage, but they said that the whole aim of this is to 'give the bowel a rest'.

Once I got home, and started to eat lightly again. So picture this: You're sitting on the couch and a massive fart comes out of the stoma. Well the first time it happened, we nearly fell around the floor with laughter, because it is such a shock! You're normally used to leaning to one side and trying to let out a 'sly one' but this thing gave the game away instantly. Totally involuntary, you would be sitting there and out comes a trumpet solo calling The Marines!

It was funny at times and you would have to do the 100m sprint to the toilet to open that clip before the whole thing burst, but at other times, it became a bit serious and disheartening. Sometimes it was really bad...

Major Gas Leak - Literally...

My dad had been along this journey with me, all the way. Ger would be my day visitor, and he would be the evening one. I was out now for a while, and was doing quite well.

He was a great man for the thought process that if you were feeling unwell or there was anything wrong with you, the best thing you could do was to go for a few pints. So my brother Gary was doing DJ at a party somewhere in town, so he arranged for him to drop the two of us into the city centre. We went into a pub called Flannery's (which is still there).

Flannery's was in a place called Temple Bar in Dublin, but at this time it wasn't a fashionable area, it was basically old bonded warehouses and grain storage type buildings for the Guinness factory nearby. Flannery's at the time was a 'semi sawdust on the floor' type pub, that could be mistaken for an old 'shebeen' but actually a legal one. Put it this way, if you asked the barman where the toilet was, he would point "that way" and hand you a toilet roll.

My dad said the reason he brought me in here was because whenever they were on strike from the FIAT factory where he worked back in the day, they would slip down to here for a few pints. The place had character. There was a table with four men sitting at it. Behind them was the dartboard. The people playing darts would literally be throwing the darts above these four men's heads as there was not much room in the pub!

So we're sitting at the bar and my dad says to the barman "do you still do the cheese and onion"? With that, the guy opens an old wooden drawer and takes out a lump of cheese, cuts it into chunks, puts it on 2 plates along with a load of onion. "Ahh this is great for you" said my dad, so I went along with it for the craic. Of course, I hadn't been used to drinking in a long time and ended up merry.

Gary picked us up and brought us home.   At about 3 am. I woke up in bed.   I could feel the bag literally bulging.   Normally in this situation, it would mean a delicate 'slide' out of the bed, staying as 'level' as I could manage, and gripping onto the circular suction thing to stop the bag coming off.   But this one was 'gonna be a gusher', so I had to act quickly.

I woke Ger beside me and said "this bag is gonna go at any second, will you get the stuff ready so we can change it"?   So it was a sidewards scramble to the bathroom.   I luckily managed to get to the toilet and empty the contents, but the circular suction thing had become loose so we had to change it.

The kids were asleep in bed.   At the time, we didn't have a proper shower but instead had a bath that you connected a shower hose onto the taps (faucets).   So I stood in the bath.

Geraldine is a 'stickler' for keeping to whatever instructions I had been given by the hospital regarding diet etc. and said the usual "how many pints did you have with your father tonight"? Of course the stereotype male answer came out "ehh only about three".

At this point I am carefully peeling the suction part off me, and she is leaning over with the shower hose trying to ease it off.

"Did you eat anything strange"? "You didn't get burgers on the way home did you"?

With that, the bag fell off and Ger got a full force splat of liquid poo smack in her face. It was everywhere. Hair, forehead, everywhere. Well... the roars out of her.   The gas from the onions was literally spraying crap everywhere! Some kids have those 'Super Soaker' water guns, it was like one of those. So the two of us ended up standing in the bath, taking turns to wash the crap off us!

It wasn't exactly a romantic moment, but I knew that after that, we would be together forever. If you're still actually reading this, take this tip: - Don't eat cheese and raw onion!

Live on stage...

I was now out of the band for a while, and they had replaced their guitarist, so it wasn't fair for me to even ask to rejoin again, so I went out on my own with my keyboard.   The keyboards were my first instrument, and I had taught myself to play the guitar, but for the moment, the guitar was retired.

I had originally got the Gypsy Rovers gig in the Airport Hotel, and they knew us very well.   The bags and the new medication were working well now so I asked the manager would she be interested in having me on a Thursday night, as a solo, as it was a quiet night, so she agreed. Later on I would get the Sunday night also.

Gypsy Rovers would play on the Friday or Saturday nights, and at the time, it was tough to see them playing without me.

I started to catch on well, and I used to play all the old slow songs at the start, and people would use the place for date nights etc. as there was a fabulous Asian restaurant in the hotel.   That eventually changed to having the place rocking with 'Simply the best' or 'Living la vida loca', I can remember at the time. Sunday nights turned into the slow night as people were just interested in winding down after the weekend.

I had 3 close people that came to the gigs all the time, my dad and two friends I had made, Tony (who has since passed away RIP) and another Brian.   They were aware of 'the bags' situation.

At the side of the stage area, I kept a briefcase. Inside the briefcase was a layout that looked like something from a James Bond movie, except this was all medical stuff!   There was tapes, spare bags, creams for sore skin, hook belts, a towel and most importantly spare trousers and shirt.

This was my emergency kit, but being in a briefcase, it looked like it could have been anything.   For musical equipment for example.

It didn't look out of place, and the three lads knew where it was, and what was in it.

The 'norm' at the time was to take a break from your gig at half time, as when the customers are so concentrated on listening to your songs, they are forgetting to buy drink, so the bar would tell you take a break mid-way.

Before half time, I was sitting at the keyboard, and I felt a 'gas bubble' sensation in the area of the bags.   I thought to myself, there is absolutely no way this thing is leaking, as I had it taped down in almost military grade style! Another 'bubble' came and I don't know what song I was singing, but the lads said later on that a shocked expression had come over my face half way through the song.

With all the bending down and standing up when you're setting up the gear, it had put strain on my 'fail safe' bag patch up job!   The problem was the half time break was ages away!   This thing was about to go, and I am on stage, in a hotel bar, with a full bag swelling!

So it was game on! I 'eye balled' the lads in the direction of the briefcase, and to follow me out to the hotel toilet. I pretended there was a small problem with the sound system and I walked ever so slowly off the stage and out to the toilet.

The problem was, the lads had had a few drinks at that time, and didn't understand what I was trying to say to them from the stage. At this point I am in the cubicle, and the bag has completely destroyed my trousers, and are soaked along with the bottom of my shirt. I am standing there for ages waiting on the lads, and no sign of them.

After a while, my dad just happened to come out to go to the toilet. "Jaysus that was a great first half" I heard as he came through the door, completely oblivious that I had been in the freezing cold cubicle for twenty minutes, in bits. It was cold, but I was sweating with both rapid dehydration and anxiety, more than likely panic also. "Get the briefcase will you"!

It was action stations literally. I had managed to get 80% of the bag poured down the toilet bowl, but the other 20% had my clothes destroyed.

So there I am telling my Dad what to pass me over the door. I stripped and wiped my whole body with special cleaning wipes. Then I got my dad to keep an eye on the door as I dried my body under the hand dryer. Then it was quickly back into the cubicle to put on a new bag. Completely lash it with tape to hold it on, change trousers and change shirt.

Nobody noticed I had a totally different shirt on. I went on and did the second half and finished the gig as if nothing had happened.

I think my Dad found a new level of respect for me that day, in the same way I always had for him. This was a different level we were on now.

The airport hotel finished for me one day when I got a crohn's pain during a performance and couldn't continue on. I was taken off by ambulance from the hotel, and Tony and Brian took down my gear, even though they didn't know how to! They put it in my car and my dad collected it the following day.

Gypsy Rovers covered my gig during that particular hospital stay, and I would cover theirs eventually, and I would get better, but it was never the same after that. I did some gigs in the hotel after that but the hotel was eventually sold, so both myself and Gypsy Rovers both lost our gigs.

Gypsy Rovers split up, and I separately retired my keyboard as I just wasn't able anymore.

A chance at CT again...

I was at home one day, and I got a call 'out of the blue' from Pat in CT again. He had a teacher, of a computer language called 'Visual Basic' who's class that he wanted me to sit in on, as that course was getting popular and their could be an opening for me.

So I was a designer and computer hardware guy, I was never a programmer. So I sat in on the class as a student and started learning and studying outside of hours separately on my own.

I was going into class one evening, and Pat called me aside and said the teacher got a full time job in Gateway 2000 and I would have to finish the course as the teacher!

I went into the class and sat down where I normally had as a student and chatted to a couple of people beside me. People started saying, "no sign of the teacher". I stood up and said "well your teacher already is here" semi in a way that you might say "Surprise". I went on to explain that I had been a student teacher and had qualified the previous week, (complete waffle, but these people had paid to do this course).

Luckily I had studied the course on my own and had figured out better ways of explaining things to people than the actual real teacher had. I would always teach by giving them the technical jargon, but following it up with a real life example where the code could be used. I was still a beginner programmer, but I was a great explainer!

I winged it and I got every single person to pass their City and Guilds Exam. I was now 'back in the door' and given the next course.

Things had been going great for a while, and I was eating anything I liked at this stage. During my sick times, I would not be able to handle eating anything spicy, or anything that contained E621 or Monosodium Glutamate on the packaging. These would give me pains and the usual symptoms as the food was going through the bowel or into the bag.

I still had my trusty briefcase with me at all times. This was always by my side.

One night I was teaching the course and the only other person in the whole building was Sharon the secretary, who was in the office across from the class room. There had been a problem with some of the screens, and several times I had to get under the tables to check cables etc. The same room was used to teach a computer assembly class, and the odd time somebody would not put them back together again correctly.

I remember reaching up to point at something on the board. When I sat down, I noticed a patch starting to form around the waist on my suit trousers. Normally I always wore black slacks and a shirt, but that day I had been for an interview and had lighter coloured suit trousers on. Nobody had noticed, they were all too busy looking at their screens.

So at the time I can remember saying to myself, "this can't be lightening striking twice" with a couple of 'F' words thrown in for good measure.   So... I grabbed the briefcase!

I slipped out the door, then passed by the closed door of the office that Sharon was in, and went down to the bathroom that was just down the stairs.

So I said to myself "calm down, this has happened before, you can deal with this"!   I checked, and the bag was coming off but had only leaked a bit, but it still had made a now very obvious patch on the front of my waist.

I realise I am using the word 'So' quite a lot in this book, but it's the only real way of explaining things in an 'as it happened' way.

Anyway, I'm now naked from the waist down, and my class are doing an exercise that I had set them, and are oblivious to what's happening.   Sharon is in her office probably doing books or class schedules or something.

I do the full cleanup operation on myself, put on the new bag, tape it up as if I am trying to stop a dam bursting, and put on my fresh clothes out of the briefcase, hoping nobody would notice I'm wearing a different colour shirt and trousers! I am finishing tucking my shirt down into my trousers, and I must have caught the bag with my hand, as 'BANG' the whole lot came off!

It is going all over my clothes again, and I am in a literal panic as I now have 'ABSOLUTELY NOTHING LEFT TO WEAR'! I am frantically trying to stop the flow but it is completely gushing out onto my trousers, completelyfrom involuntarily.

I am racking my brain trying to figure out a solution, but there was none.

I did the cleanup routine again from the kit in the briefcase. I remember feeling possibly the lowest I had ever felt. I think I can actually acknowledge that this was my all time low. Sorry to you readers, but real is real.

I remember gathering up all of my stuff from the toilet and walking down the stairs of the building in my underpants.   I was lucky the rest of the building was empty.   I walked down to the back yard where my car was parked, got in and started to drive home.

Meanwhile Sharon and the class were still there and were not aware of anything!   I had to phone Sharon from the car, and tell her I had got sick with a pain in my side, and went home.   She was shocked, as she was now going to have to go into a class and tell them the teacher is gone and the class is over.

I had no cigarettes in the car.   I remember pulling into a petrol station and pulling up near to the door.   I couldn't get out of the car, so I actually lied to a guy going by saying that I'm in a wheelchair, and could he take this money and get me 20 smokes!   Yes, I felt that bad. That was the last ever class that I taught in CT, and they never knew what really happened. Until now I suppose!

The Reversal and Removal...

By the end of about six or seven months, the hospital knew that I wasn't coping with the bags.   It's not that I wasn't coping with the bags themselves, as I quickly got used to them.

In my case it was where they had placed them, on a crease in my body, that would have been fine if I was laying down all the time, but any sort of bending at all and there was a risk.

I was a very 'public' person.   I dealt face to face with customers, I sang in front of crowds, I taught classes, if I didn't do this kind of stuff, then it probably would have been a different story.   Added to that, the circular area of skin around my stoma was now really badly inflamed due to changing the bags so often, and using fabric nursing tape to bind myself like a 'mummy from Egypt' didn't help things.

My surgeon team decided it was time to reverse the bags operation, and after another surgery, I had no bags.

Of course they went through the same scar again, and I remember saying to them at the time that they should install a zip to make it easier.

The physician team also switched me onto a new drug called Entocort.

The one redeeming quality that made these months of chaos worthwhile was that the bags worked!

That's why at the start of this, I said if it was to come for me again, I would handle it totally differently. The bags gave my bowel a rest. It bypassed the 'inflamed area of tube' and brought 'your stuff' out to an easy empty bag – if you behaved yourself!

I don't think I 'fully behaved myself' at the time. Before the bags I couldn't eat hardly anything, especially my beloved Chinese food, but when the bags came on and the inflamed bit was bypassed, then it was anything goes!

I was ecstatic at the time of the ability to have

a curry and not be 'dying' after it! I probably had too much of that kind of stuff as coming home from a gig late at night, I would pop in to the Chinese takeaway and get some 'Chicken Chow Mein' and eat it before I got home. Ger would be going mad when the bag would start bubbling and filling up in the bed. I would be sprinting out to the toilet like 'Usain Bolt', and she would be roaring "did you have anything to eat on the way home" and of course I would say "No, nothing at all". Then you'd hear "are you sure..."?

I remember getting a turn against sweetcorn. It wasn't that I was allergic to it or anything like that, it was because sweetcorn doesn't seem to dissolve much, so it would look the same way it came out in the bag, as when it went in after eating it! So it put me off it for years!

But after the reversal, the combination of the bowel rest and the Entocort actually went on to give me a good few years of a break. I was starting to feel 'normal' again.

I was learning that this condition will give you 'up and down times' so we used to grab the good times, and persevere with the bad times.

Good times we would bring the kids on a day out or a holiday, bad times were usually doing pain management, but we got through, and we kept the kids away from this stuff, as much as we could.

But now we were starting to manage, but it would be a long road ahead, always knowing it would be a 'never ending road', but this time, better able to handle it.   I remember myself and Geraldine saying to each other, that if we could handle all this, then we could handle anything.

The Comeback Kid Rides Again…

So now I have a young family, I'm just out of hospital, have no job of any kind, I weigh about eight stone, and I haven't got a bean.

I remember having no clothes as they were now all too big for me, so it meant I had to go up to the local welfare officer, who was in the local clinic at the time, and ask him for money for a track suit or something as I had nothing to wear.

There were some people in the queue to go into him that were 'chancing' their arm, pretending they needed money for this and that, but in reality one of their mates had got something, and she tipped off this one what to say and what to ask for. You used to be able to hear the swearing and language, when they'd get turned down, as she walked out of the room in her 'Air Jordans' that were very expensive shoes at the time, her child in the pram had a matching pair!

When he saw me, he looked as if he got a bit of a fright, as I looked a bit skeletal! I asked him for the clothes, and he not only did that, he got us a washing machine, as ours was getting repaired all the time. He stuck close with me over the coming months, and got me through. I'll never forget him for that.

Shortly after that I was collecting the kids from the local school, and their teacher Mrs. B came out to me and knowing I was recovering from an operation, asked me could I do her a favor, and teach her class computers, as it wasn't really her thing. I would be helping her out, and she would be helping me out. I personally think she was doing me the bigger favor, and wanted to try and see me get going again – good on you Mrs. B.

I worked with my now good friends Joe and Rory, and I got the computer room setup. The kids were loving it. I got some money from the parents committee and we bought two giant televisions, one at each end of the room, and rigged them up to my main screen. We now had a digital blackboard, before any other school in the area had one!

Within a month, almost all of the other teachers asked me to do their classes, so I made a rota, and every kid from first class up got 40 minutes a week. It was brilliant, because we weren't doing boring stuff, we were doing typing lessons, brain training puzzles and games, digital comics with a digital camera, and even stop motion animation. We were way ahead of our time as the curriculum at the time had nothing in place. Do you remember the teacher would send somebody down for the projector, and come back with big roll of slide film? Well half them would be so scratched, you couldn't see them, so I scanned them and turned them into digital form and put them on video for the teacher. It was a thrill to be doing all this.

But, I needed money of some kind, so it turned out that I was going to be able to do this through the Irish training board FAS. So I had started in FAS a good few years and now back in it! I ended up staying there for three more years, and in that time I got donations of decent computers from a large insurance company that were changing their systems. I was really 'up' now at this time, and I was able to replace every single computer in the computer room, and also one on each teacher's desk. When your mind is 'up', your body is also 'up'.

After a while, opportunity knocked. Parents were starting to come into me and say stuff like, oh my little Robert loves your class etc., but then would follow it immediately with a question how to fix her computer in the house. I would say, sure bring it over, and I would fix it during classes. After a while I noticed a pile of computers lined up in a queue beside me. I thought...hang on...there could be a business in this! I decided to 'grab the bull by the horns' and take a chance.

Over in FAS the attendees were meant to do courses, but nobody was taking up the ones that were being offered, so I jumped on the chance, when Meg H offered me a Start you own business course up in the Enterprise Centre in Navan nearby.

It was an excellent course, and I was so enthusiastic, I ended up being a stand in teacher sometimes, introducing companies to E-Commerce, which was only beginning to happen at that time.

So in 2003, I registered my computer repair company Ashbourne PC. Some of those kids I thought went on to do huge things. I still see some of them when I fix their computers in their homes, and one of the main things they said gives them a benefit in work is the fact that I had taught them to touch type. Most people use their index fingers! I went on to teach 'gap year' students for a period in the secondary school, but the school days and FAS ended shortly after. I was independent again!

I later subcontracted for DELL for a couple of years, travelling Ireland, replacing screens, laptop motherboards and more. With the bags gone and the entocort, we got about 10 years without major surgery.

'Normal time' was spent doing pain management, getting the odd set back, and then pain management again. Sometimes it would be the cause of dehydration as the length of my bowel was getting shorter with each piece that they snipped away, so I would have the setback, and they would take me in for a few days, put me on a drip, and then out again.

Sometimes it could be down to my weak immune system. One time, the kids got Chicken Pox, which is nasty at any age, but when they transferred it to me, it went everywhere. I had sores all over my body, even my eye lids! I was kept in isolation for about 10 days. I was so contagious, that the staff would open the door with the early type of PPE gear, and when leaving would put a big yellow X made out of hazard tape of my door.

But to myself and Ger, these were only hiccups to us at this stage, as we had 'seen it all' by now.

One of these 'hiccups' actually turned out to be a blessing, when somebody close to me had a cold, and gave it to me.   Mine turned into pneumonia, and again I was carted into the emergency room.   While I was there they had me on a drip stabilising me as my lungs were filling with fluid.   Of course all I am thinking about is going out the back for a smoke!   With Pneumonia!

Regardless, I went out and lit up the smoke, and tried to smoke it.   I nearly passed out as I had no air.   I came back into the room and said to the nurse to "take the cigarettes and lighter out of my pocket and put them into the sharps bin (the one for used needles)".   I did this so I could not go in after them.   My smoking days were over.   It had taken 30 years...

The Remission...

Remission is the word they use for the 'good' periods in between your 'bad active times' with Crohn's.   My remission periods were getting longer, and my 'active' times were getting less frequent.

At the time of writing there's no cure for Crohn's disease, but I firmly believe that my acceptance of it, my mindset about it, and the apprenticeship of disastrous things I had gone through with it, had helped me.   The doctors were also 'upbeat' about the new medications that were coming along.

There came a time period where rather than having a Crohn's mass, I would have the odd flares from time to time, but mainly with Crohn's related type of things.   Dehydration, Hernias, Blood Infections (from a piece of 'gauze bandage' being left inside me after an operation) and other things like that but no major surgery.   They call this stage 'deep remission'.   It can go on for years.   I got ten...

The Final Fling...so far!

So I was still sub-contracting for Dell and was going great. I loved the job, as it came naturally to me, and I loved the fact that every day was a different person and a different place. I am feeling great or 'I think I am'...

What did I do? Once I started feeling in top form, I started taking on extra 'runs' that the full time staff were turning down, as the difference was, they got paid by the day so tried to do as little as possible, as they were getting the same wage regardless. However I was a contractor and was getting paid per individual fix job.

Sometimes I would arrive in a Government office, and there would be five computers lined up to change the motherboards, which just popped out. Even though this was one building, I was getting paid for five jobs, the same as five individual buildings. Dell had supplied some Government departments with a model of computer that developed a small fault, and Dell wanted every single one to be fixed by replacing the motherboard. Garda stations, Hospitals, Army, and all Civil Service for example. It was a 'gravy train', during the boom time, pre the property crash of 2008.

Pat from CT was setting up his own computer shop at the time, and I was delighted to be able to give a bit of 'payback' by getting him in on the 'gravy train' as they wanted more contract staff. So this helped him get setup. I'm a massive believer in Karma and it was great to send some in his direction.

Unfortunately... I went back to my old ways of panicking about 'how long will this contract last' and taking double the amount of jobs others were taking. Problem was that the company loved me because I was doing them all correctly and getting great ratings surveys.

But it went crazy. I took on a contract for 6 months, driving from Ashbourne Meath, up to Belfast in Northern Ireland every day, then across a mountain range to Omagh and

Enniskillen, and then drive back home in heavy traffic.   Every day for 6 months.

My side was beginning to give me the warning signals, the dull pain, and the pain when food was going through your intestine.   I was eating 'on the road' and drinking at minimum 10 cups of coffee a day.   Wasn't really a good diet...

One night in bed, we had the good old Déjà vu again.   This time it was a blockage, and I was doubled up in pain on the floor.   It was a by now 'usual case' of blue lights flashing outside of Brian and Ger's house, and the ambulance men struggling to bring me down the stairs on the stretcher as my knees are up to my chest with the pain, and if I try to move, it makes it worse.   I have to say, I have the best neighbours in the world, but I think we would have woken them at 4 am. Many times!

Luckily the hospital 'on duty' that night was Blanchardstown Hospital, and this proved to be the beginning of a series of events that have kept me here to write this book!

By now, Geraldine had learned to drive, and this hospital was 25 minutes away from my home, so it would be easier than the old days. The best thing was, they had a great Crohn's team.   I had 'got away with' a break of about 10 years from surgery after the bags, so my mindset going in here was more 'mature'.

To cut a long story short, they did all the usual tests and added new one like the MRI scan to make sure, but they discovered that a large piece of bowel would have to come out, as it was badly inflamed and had holes in it.   When a piece of bowel narrows, it can stick to the other side and it is then, we will say, 'kinked'.

But then if a piece of food manages to go through, it can 'rip' the stuck piece off the inner wall and take a lump of opposite wall with it forming a hole!   So you can't have your 'poop' leaking into your main body system, so it's got to come out.

The week before surgery, the surgeon had told me that he would have to give me bags again, and this at the time, disappointed me a lot, but I was accepting it.

A couple of nights before the operation, I couldn't sleep. Down in the lobby of the hospital, they have a vending machine for tea, so I went down and got one. I then decided to go into the Oratory. For those who don't know, an oratory is like a small church. It's not a catholic or a protestant thing, it's purely intended as a place of prayer.

I said a little personal prayer, and hoped for the best for my operation. There was a podium there that a celebrant would use to stand at and it had a wooden cross on it. I don't know why I decided to go over and touch the cross, but as soon as I did, I felt the exact same 'magnetic' type sensation that I had felt all those years before. Of course, I was frightened out of my skin, as it was 2 a.m. and nobody around, but I recognised the feeling, and I got the thought going through my head, that 'everything was going to be ok'.

It turned out, the night of my surgery, the surgeon that was originally meant to do my surgery had to go somewhere, and my operation was done by the 'stand in' surgeon!

He didn't give me bags, he said he got around it somehow. They did, however, take a large bit out, and of course, went in via the same scar!

They did another MRI after the operation and were able to measure the length of small bowel I have left in my body. You normally have about 22 feet. I have now only got 10 left.

Apparently you can live with around 5, but heavily medicated. So in my case, if ever I do need surgery again (touch wood) I will gladly accept the bags and be delighted I have the option of them! Total turnaround!

Prevention is better than cure...

The new 'physician' doctors in Blanchardstown wanted to change me to a new drug.   They wanted to give it to me before the surgery, but it was too late at that stage to start it then.   I had heard of this drug before, but never really looked into it.   This drug was Humira.

This drug seemed to be way ahead of the others.   At the time, they even had their own 'Humira Nurse' in the hospital.   You were given a 'welcome pack' with this drug, similar to what you would be given at a conference, leather folder, professional documentation, the lot!   I have since found out, that this drug is very expensive, so I wasn't surprised with the highly professional approach.   The packaging said something similar to 'welcome to the rest of your life'.

As I said at the start of the book, everybody is different, and different drugs will work for different people, and won't for others.

This one worked for me (so far).   It is an 'injection pen' that you give yourself.   It's not like a needle, its more like a cartridge, that give you a little sting. I take it every 2 weeks. It is encouraged that you make a YouTube video of yourself, giving your first injection so you can look back on it. Mine is still there, and at the time of writing, was 9 years ago.

It is brilliant, and you will eventually find a drug that works for you, but I firmly believe that if I didn't change all the mental things, it may not have worked.

When I talk to people with Crohn's, Colitis, or IBS, you will find we all have a common denominator – we are 'people pleasers'. We like to be organized, we like to do the job right, we hate to let anybody down. We do more than what is expected of us, and unfortunately some people are taken advantage of in that way, then it's out of sight, out of mind.

I had to learn that if I don't want to 'let people down' for example, I have to do certain things to keep out of hospital. If I am lying on a hospital bed, staring at the tiled ceiling all day,

I am no use to the company then, am I? I am no use to my family. I am no use to my body, because us 'Crohnies' come in 2 parts, our minds, and our bodies.

In our case, our mind reckons we are well able to take on certain things, at a certain speed, and get a certain reward. But our body is saying – ehhhh NO! "You're starting to put me under a bit of strain here Brian, so you're gonna have to figure out a solution".

Well it took me a lot of years, multiple operations, probably a wrestler's bodyweight in tablets, and untold grief, but I finally found the solution... the ability to say "F..k it"!

Now you won't find that in any medical book, and I can't even put the full word here as it might change the age restriction of the book, but the solution really is to learn to say "F..k it", but in your head only, as obviously I don't want hundreds of people going around shouting "F..k it" at the top of their voice.

I will explain.

If you want to stay well, you will have to learn:

• If you can't do anything about something, even though you've tried your best, just leave it, and maybe try again tomorrow. "Oh but it can't wait until tomorrow" I hear you say... Yes it CAN, as if you end up on a hospital bed tonight, it won't get done anyway! See what I mean? Learn to say F..k it! From now on we will verbally replace that with 'Let it go'. Keep singing that song from 'Frozen The Movie'!

• Your boss is hassling you with a deadline. It MUST be done today. You are dependent on other people to, for example, provide supplies, provide knowledge, do a different part of the job. You are starting to feel a familiar tension and pain in your stomach area. If this scenario is a regular thing in your job, then either change job, or get the people you are dependent upon to pull their weight, and stop doing it all yourself, like you usually do!

You say: "Oh but I can't change job, I won't get another one".   Yes you will, especially if you start secretly applying while you're in the troublesome one to give yourself an edge. You will find that the tension will be less, because you now know you're getting 'out of there'!

If you can't find something in the same industry, then switch to a different industry.   I have had to change at least 5 times.   Started as a salesman, then printer, then teacher, then graphic designer, then computer repair and web company.   <u>The main thing you need to understand is that you won't be able to do ANY job if you're flat on your back, because you didn't acknowledge the warning signs your body was giving to you</u>.   'Let it go'!

• Avoid negative people.   You might have a friend, a relative, a workmate that is just constantly negative.   They never have a good word to say.   You love your job, but they come in to work moaning about the hours, the pay, how tired they are after being out drinking the night before.   The 'can't wait to finish' people. I'm not saying you have to live in a world where nothing goes wrong, but these type of people give off a massive amount of 'negative energy' and this can bring YOU down, so avoid, or just get rid.   'Let it go'!

• Avoid 'Completely un-trained medical experts on Crohn's and it's medications!   I have been totally honest right from the start that I am not medically trained, and everything you read here is my own personal experience and opinions.   But there is an absolute army of keyboard warriors on the internet, that write stuff claiming to be fact, when it's completely unproved lies.   They rubbish certain medicines and treatments, just because 'it didn't work for them', but in reality it has worked for plenty of other people, and this person just needs to keep going until their doctor finds the right one, that works for THEM.   The problem is, vulnerable people swallow everything these people and web sites say, and spread 'the facts' to others, and suddenly there is a large amount of people around the world not taking their prescribed medication.

In the early days, I fell for this stupidity but soon 'copped on'. When you are desperate, you will 'clutch at anything' that will give you a break.

So I think it's time to stop mentally saying 'the word that rhymes with book it' and realise that in my own personal opinion, and I stress that this is my own person opinion, the whole idea is about 'taking control of BOTH your mind AND your body, as at the end of the day, you are responsible for both.

Doctors and medication will help you, but at the end of the day, if you don't change both your way of thinking, AND your way of acting, you will be delaying your chances of getting well.

You need to finally come to the realisation that YOU come first, above EVERYTHING and

EVERYBODY, because if you are not well on a hospital bed, YOU can't be there for the people you LOVE.   So by addressing the causes first, and then slowly getting rid of them, one at a time, then your medication has a chance to work.   It took a long time, but this is what eventually worked for me.

There are plenty of support mechanisms to get you through this stage.   I can only really refer to Ireland, but whatever country you are living in, I am confident, that if you look, you will find them.   Examples in Ireland were at the time:

• The ability to take a Mortgage Break.   If you are at rock bottom, or near to it, just go and tell the truth to your bank.   Banks don't necessarily spend all their days trying to repossess houses, if the person is genuinely trying to make an effort to save it.   They are in the business of making money, so if they can give you a break for a year, they will still make money on all the other years you will be paying interest.   We were able to get a mortgage break of a year at the time, and it gave me the time to get back on my feet.

• Back to work Enterprise Allowance Scheme. When I left the schools and setup the business, you were able to keep your welfare entitlements for a couple of years, to help you get on your feet.

There are plenty of these type of support mechanisms, and you will find them if you do your research, or if you talk to other people who have gone through the same thing as you.

Another main person is your local Doctor. I was extremely lucky to have 2 amazing local doctors, Dr. P and in later years Dr. M. Dr. P spent endless hours coming to my house during the bad times, and had the patience of a saint. I will always be forever in his debt. Dr. M was great at all the new treatments and put me onto Ensure Plus, which was a game changer for quickly putting on weight after an operation when I couldn't eat anything else.

• Listen especially to your main specialist in the hospital.   When he or she is doing their rounds with their 'minions', they tend not to have time to talk directly to you.   INTERRUPT them and point at one of the 'minions' and say to the specialist, "Sorry for interrupting Doctor, but later on can you send this guy back to me, and get him to explain to me in simple plain English, what an extended right hemicolectomy is, and what is the exact procedure you guys will be doing on me?   I used to do that, and it worked.   The specialist gets to know you then, and you will find that next time he talks directly to you!

But of course my total saviour was and is my wife Geraldine, who I know, hand on heart, I wouldn't be here today if it wasn't for her.   For you the reader, try to have somebody like this. You will need help at times, and never be too proud to accept it.   At the end of the day, sometimes you will just have accept outside help, and learn to say "F...." ahh hang on, let's not start that again!

We're gonna need a bigger file!

And so began my new relationship with Blanchardstown Hospital. The same medical file that had started in The Richmond, moved to Beaumount, transferred to St. Vincents, with the occasional transfer to the Mater, had now ended up in Connolly Hospital Blanchardstown. It is now the size of 3 Yellow Pages, and is still growing!

So I was reminded of the famous line in 'Jaws The Movie' – "I think we're gonna need a bigger boat", well I can tell you, we are definitely gonna need a bigger file!

Due to the physical size of this file, and the tattered appearance of it from being sent everywhere, I notice that junior and senior doctors take a particular interest in me.   I always seem to get appointments quickly, and get really well looked after.   It's possibly because each department wants to see who is this guy!

When I go for appointments, all the different patients files are laid out on a trolley.   Mine is HUGE, so the junior doctors always want to have a 'flick' through it, and I get called.   I suppose it's a strange way of thinking, that I'm glad I get seen to at clinics really quickly because I have had all these things done to me and it's taken so much paperwork!

I think I have used up 7 trees from the Amazon at this point!

Good times are here again...

If you're still here, I have to congratulate you. It wasn't really an easy book for you to read, but Crohn's Disease isn't an easy condition to live with, but what I want you to take from this book is that it CAN be lived with.

After the last operation and the new drug, things started to go good again for me.

At age 50, I went to college and did a Degree in Digital Technology and Design.   When I left school, I had qualified to get into the College of Marketing and Design on Parnell St. Dublin, but the funds just were not there at the time.   I was delighted to have my parents at that graduation.   I will never forget the pride on their faces, as the ceremony was in St. Patrick's Cathedral, and it was like being at Hogwarts!

I had always wanted to have a degree, but I didn't necessarily need one.   The whole thing was a personal journey, and the fact that 'I could still some ass with the rest of them'!

The same year, I must have been on a roll, as I got the band back together! The exact same original lineup as all those years ago, myself, Jimmy C and Martin F. We had our first practice in about 20 years, and it was like we had never gone away. We still play together today!

We are almost finished here. In later years, I had massive open heart surgery, but that would need another book. The only thing I can tell you, is the day before the operation, a nurse was shaving my chest. There was a curtain with a wall behind it at the side of my bed. The nurse suddenly turned around and said 'oh sorry' to the person he had bumped into behind him, as he was rushing. When he turned around, there was nobody there, and he said "hmm that's strange, I could have sworn I just bumped into somebody there".

I looked down, and at the end of my bed was my father in law Tommy, who I had become close to when I was visiting him in the nursing home, before he died. I wasn't on any medication or pre medication. It wasn't a flash moment, he was there for a couple of seconds, and was watching the nurse shaving me and smiling. I went into that heart operation without a care in the world. I really had no fear about it, even though it was the most dangerous one I was ever going to have.

The condition I had was most likely an inherited genetic one, where the central wall of my heart was growing wider, and was slowly closing down one of my 4 chambers. You read about this a lot, when you see athletes or footballers dying suddenly during the game.

The surgeon only did about 3 of these a year, and I got chosen as one of them. He said after the operation that he reckoned with the rate of growth, that I only had about 12 weeks left. So I reckon Tommy brought me luck that time.

But again, due to the fact that I had changed my thinking, for me, it was a non-event. It was extremely serious, but I was so relaxed about it, I feel I literally sailed through it. This is a long way from the 'original me'.

I hope you have enjoyed my story. People who know me will tell you I am now probably the most chilled person you will ever come across, especially in crisis situations.

I still like to be efficient, and am still highly organised, but am able to do things in a completely different way than before. The main thing is that I have learned to spot the warning signals, your body will tell you.

The icing on the cake for me would be if I knew, somebody, somewhere around the world, used something they spotted in the book, and started feeling a bit better because of it.

If you're a 'newbie', don't be frightened, not ALL of this is going to happen to you, just because it happened to me! Things have changed, technology and medicine have now advanced and are still advancing.

Just remember...

You don't feel pain when you're laughing.

You can choose to either laugh or cry.

I choose to laugh!   Laugh along with me!

"Let it go!"

Best of luck – Your Fellow 'Old Crohnie' - Brian